Smart Keto Vegetarian Recipes

Fast, Delicious and Affordable High-Fat Recipes for a Plant-Based Ketogenic Diet

Lidia Wong

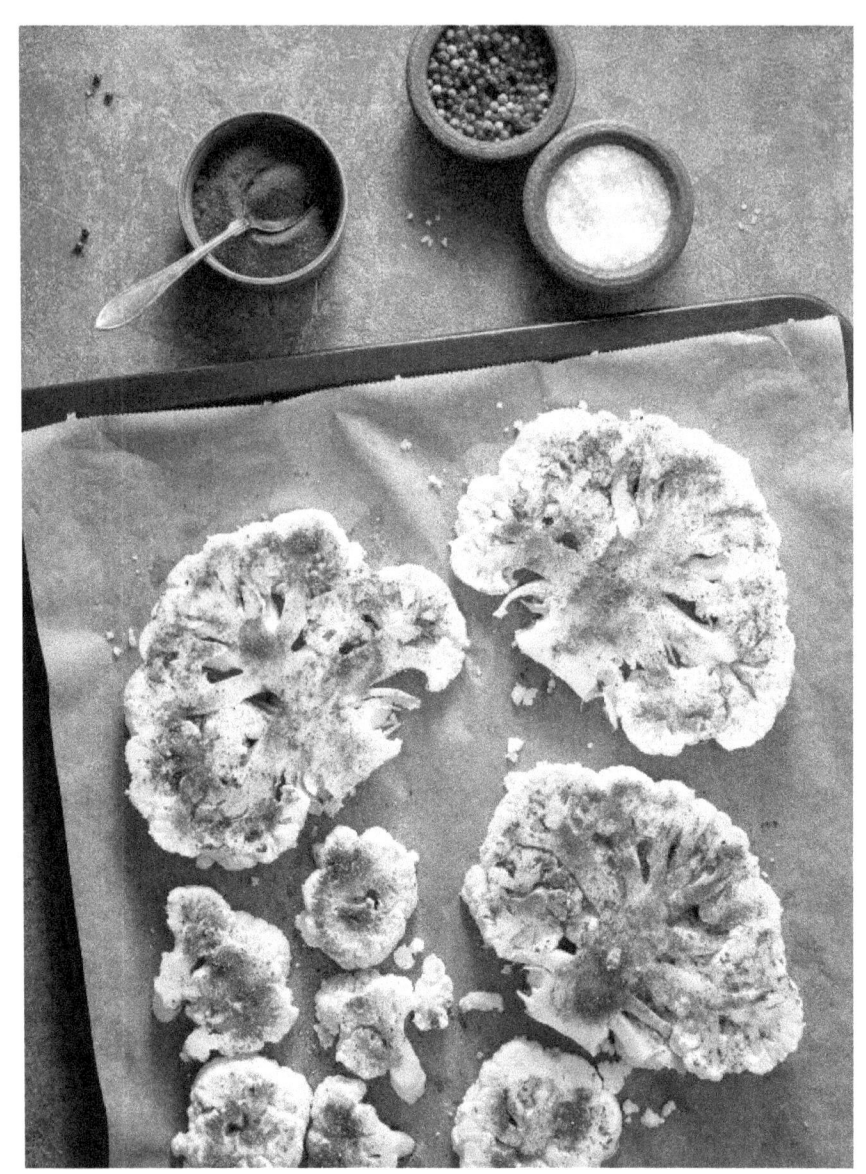

© **Copyright 2021 by Lidia Wong - All rights reserved.**

The content contained within this book may not be reproduced, duplicated or transmitted without direct written permission from the author or the publisher.
Under no circumstances will any blame or legal responsibility be held against the publisher, or author, for any damages, reparation, or monetary loss due to the information contained within this book. Either directly or indirectly.

Legal Notice:
This book is copyright protected. This book is only for personal use. You cannot amend, distribute, sell, use, quote or paraphrase any part, or the content within this book, without the consent of the author or publisher.

Disclaimer Notice:
Please note the information contained within this document is for educational and entertainment purposes only. All effort has been executed to present accurate, up to date, and reliable, complete information. No warranties of any kind are declared or implied. Readers acknowledge that the author is not engaging in the rendering of legal, financial, medical or professional advice. The content within this book has been derived from various sources. Please consult a licensed professional before attempting any techniques outlined in this book.
By reading this document, the reader agrees that under no circumstances is the author responsible for any losses, direct or indirect, which are incurred as a result of the use of information contained within this document, including, but not limited to, — errors, omissions, or inaccuracies.

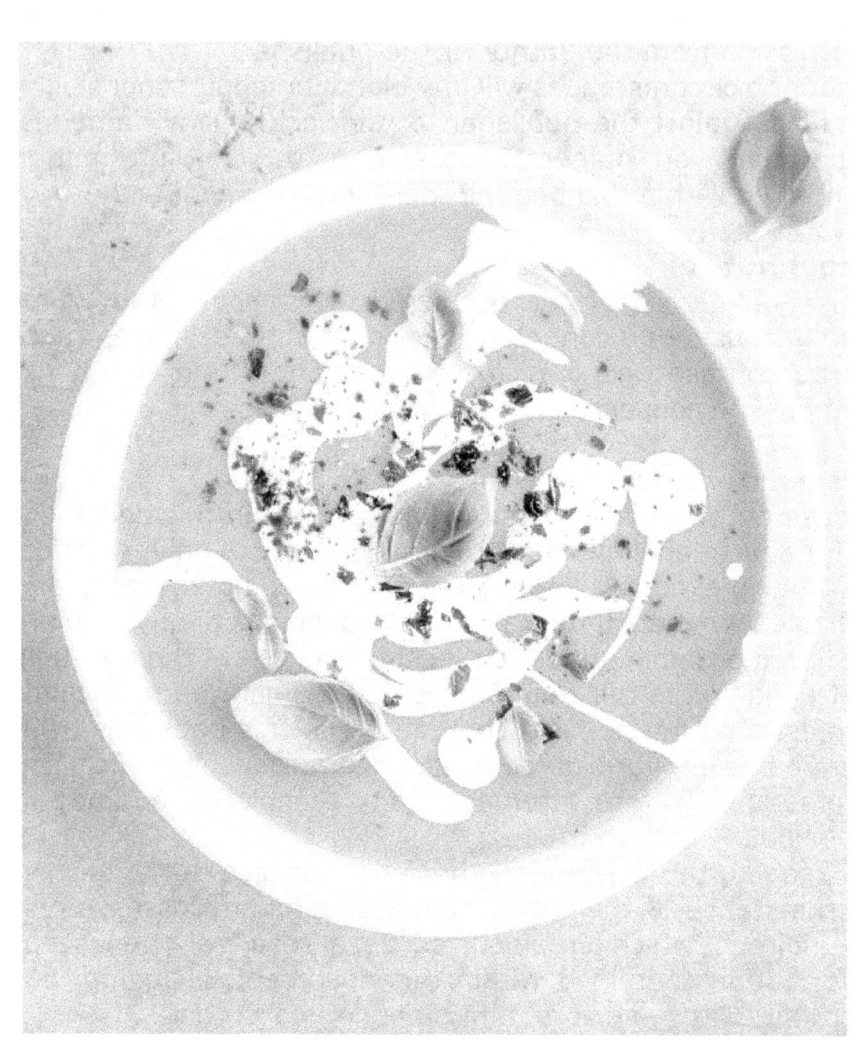

TABLE OF CONTENTS

INTRODUCTION 1

Avocado Spinach Cucumber Breakfast Smoothie 3

Green Beans and Radishes Bake 4

Arugula and Artichokes Bowls 6

Avocado, Pine Nuts and Chard Salad 7

Cinnamon Cauliflower Rice, Zucchinis and Spinach . 9

Asparagus, Bok Choy and Radish Mix 11

Roasted Cauliflower and Broccoli 12

Mexican Vegan Mince 14

Chili-Garlic Edamame 16

Arugula Mushroom Salad 18

Spicy Cheese with Tofu Balls 20

Cucumber and Cauliflower Mix 22

Bell Pepper Sauté 24

Wild Rice Mix 26

Squash And Spinach Mix 28

Baked Artichokes and Green Beans 30

Herbed Risotto 32

Braised Cabbage And Apples 34

Eggplant and Garlic Sauce 36

Warm Watercress Mix 38

Purple Carrot Mix 40

Broccoli, Garlic, and Rigatoni 42

Broccoli Stew 44

Arugula Salad 46

Catalan-style Greens 48

White And Wild Mushroom Barley Soup 50

Thai-Inspired Coconut Soup 52

Tofu Avocado Keto Noodles 54

Crunchy Cauliflower Bites 56

Broccoli and Almonds 58

Twice Baked Spaghetti Squash 59

Spicy Jalapeno Brussels sprouts 62

Risotto Bites 63

Jicama and Guacamole 65

Black Sesame Wonton Chips 67

Peppers and Hummus 68

Crispy Brussels Sprouts 70

Coconut Bites 72

Spiced Okra Bites 74

Chaffle Cannoli 76

Mango Coconut Cream Pie 78

Lime in the Coconut Chia Pudding 81

Grapefruit Cream 83

Chia Bars 84

Fudgy Chocolate Cake 86

Baked Apples. 89

Cream Cheese Cookies 91

Yogurt Smoothie with Cinnamon and Mango 93

Cocoa Peach Cream 95

Minty Almond Cups 96

Lime Cake 97

Berry Cream 99

NOTE **101**

INTRODUCTION

The keto diet is the shortened term for ketogenic diet and it is essentially a high-fat and low-carb diet that helps you lose weight, thereby bringing various health benefits. This diet drastically restricts your carb intake while increasing your fat intake; this pushes your body to go into a state know as "*ketosis*". We will tackle ketosis in a bit.

The human body uses glucose from carbs to fuel metabolic pathways—meaning various bodily functions like digestion, breathing, etc.. Essentially, anything that needs energy. Even when you are resting, the body needs fuel or energy for you to continue living. If you think about it, when have you ever stopped breathing, or your heart stopped beating, or your liver stopped from cleansing the body, or your kidneys from filtering blood?

Never, unless you're dead, which is the only time in which the body doesn't need energy. In normal circumstances, glucose is the primary pathway when it comes to sourcing the body's energy.

But the body also has another pathway; it can utilize fats to fuel the various bodily processes. And this is what we call "*ketosis*". And the body can only enter ketosis when there is no glucose available, thus the reason for sticking to a low-carb diet is essential in the keto diet. Since no glucose is available, the body is pushed to use fats—it can either come from the food you consume or from your body's fat reserves—the adipose tissue or from the flabby parts of your body. This is how the keto diet helps you lose weight, by burning up all those stored fats that you have and using it to fuel bodily processes.

That said, if for whatever reason you are a vegetarian, following a ketogenic diet can be extremely difficult. A vegetarian diet is largely free of animal products, which means that food tends to be usually high in carbohydrates. Still, with careful planning, it is possible. This Cookbook will provide you with various easy and delicious dishes to help you stick to your ketogenic diet plan while being a vegetarian.

Enjoy!

Avocado Spinach Cucumber Breakfast Smoothie

Preparation Time: 10 minutes

Servings: 1

Ingredients:

- 1-ounce spinach, fresh, chopped
- 1.8-ounces cucumber, chopped
- 1 scoop protein powder
- 1 ½ cups almond milk
- 1.8-ounce celery, chopped
- 1.8-ounce avocado
- 1 tablespoon coconut oil
- 10 drops liquid Stevia

Directions:

1. Add all the ingredients into a blender and blend until smooth. Serve and enjoy!

Nutritional Values (Per Serving):

Calories: 385 Fat: 26.6 g Carbohydrates: 12.9 g
Sugar: 2.7 g Protein: 26.1 g Cholesterol: 65 mg

Green Beans and Radishes Bake

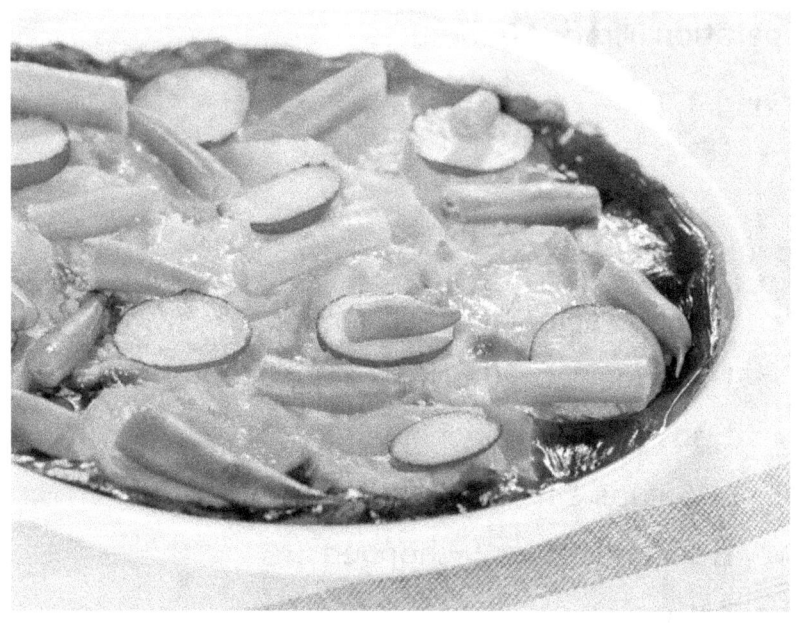

Preparation time: 10 minutes

Cooking time: 25 minutes

Servings: 4

Ingredients:

- 2 tablespoons olive oil
- 2 cups radishes, sliced
- 1 pound green beans, trimmed and halved
- 1 cup coconut cream

- 1 teaspoon sweet paprika
- 1 cup cashew cheese, shredded
- Salt and black pepper to the taste
- 1 tablespoon chives, chopped

Directions:

1. In a roasting pan, combine the green beans with the radishes and the other ingredients except for the cheese and toss.
2. Sprinkle the cheese on top, introduce in the oven at 375 degrees F and bake for 25 minutes.
3. Divide the mix between plates and serve.

Nutrition:

calories 130, fat 1, fiber 0.4, carbs 1, protein 0.1

Arugula and Artichokes Bowls

Preparation time: 5 minutes

Cooking time: 0 minutes

Servings: 4

Ingredients:

- 1 cup canned artichoke hearts, drained and quartered
- 2 cups baby arugula
- ¼ cup walnuts, chopped
- 1 tablespoon balsamic vinegar
- 2 tablespoons cilantro, chopped
- 2 tablespoons olive oil
- Salt and black pepper to the taste
- 1 tablespoon lemon juice

Directions:

1. In a bowl, combine the artichokes with the arugula, walnuts and the other ingredients, toss, divide into smaller bowls and serve for lunch.

Nutrition:

calories 200, fat 2, fiber 1, carbs 5, protein 7

Avocado, Pine Nuts and Chard Salad

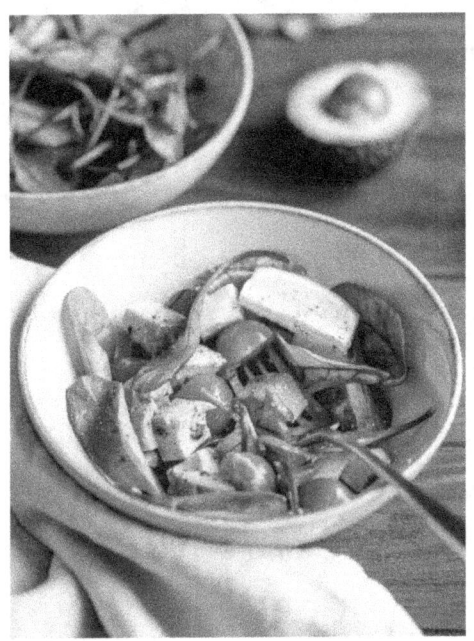

Preparation time: 5 minutes

Cooking time: 15 minutes

Servings: 4

Ingredients:

- 1 pound Swiss chard, roughly chopped
- 1 avocado, peeled, pitted and roughly cubed
- 2 tablespoons olive oil

- ¼ cup pine nuts, toasted
- 2 spring onions, chopped
- 1 tablespoon balsamic vinegar
- Salt and black pepper to the taste

Directions:

1. Heat up a pan with the oil over medium heat, add the spring onions, pine nuts and the chard, stir and sauté for 5 minutes.
2. Add the vinegar and the other ingredients, toss, cook over medium heat for 10 minutes more, divide into bowls and serve for lunch.

Nutrition:

calories 120, fat 2, fiber 1, carbs 4, protein 8

Cinnamon Cauliflower Rice, Zucchinis and Spinach

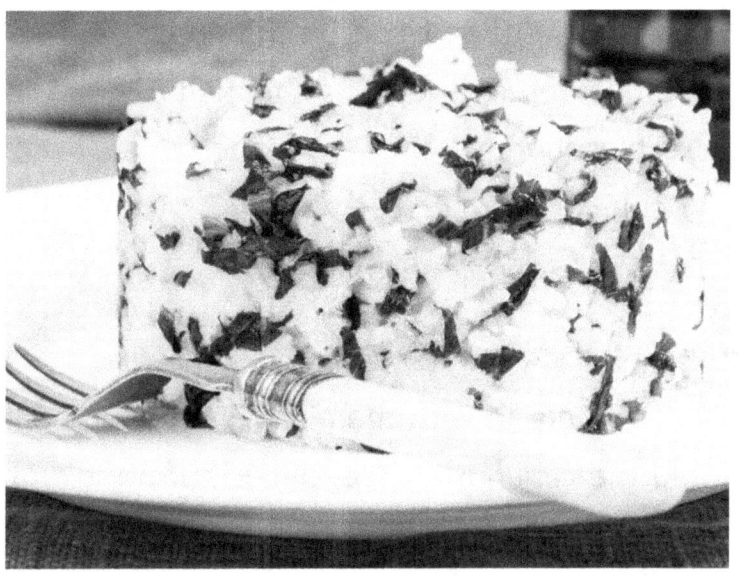

Preparation time: 10 minutes

Cooking time: 10 minutes

Servings: 4

Ingredients:

- 1 cup cauliflower rice
- 1 zucchini, sliced
- 1 cup baby spinach

- 2 tablespoons olive oil
- ½ cup veggie stock
- ½ teaspoon turmeric powder
- ¼ teaspoon cinnamon powder
- A pinch of sea salt and black pepper
- 1/3 cup dates, dried and chopped
- 1 tablespoon almonds, chopped
- ¼ cup chives, chopped

Directions:

1. Heat up a pan with the oil over medium heat, add the cauliflower rice, dates, turmeric and cinnamon and sauté for 3 minutes.
2. Add the zucchini and the other ingredients, toss, cook the mix for 7 minutes more, divide between plates and serve.

Nutrition:

calories 189, fat 2, fiber 2, carbs 20, protein 7

Asparagus, Bok Choy and Radish Mix

Preparation time: 10 minutes

Cooking time: 12 minutes

Servings: 4

Ingredients:

- ½ pound asparagus, trimmed and halved
- 1 cup bok choy, torn
- 1 cup radishes, halved
- 2 tablespoons balsamic vinegar
- 2 tablespoons olive oil
- 2 teaspoon Italian seasoning
- 2 teaspoons garlic powder
- 1 teaspoon coriander, ground
- 1 teaspoon fennel seeds, crushed
- 1 tablespoon chives, chopped

Directions:

1. Heat up a pan with the oil over medium heat, add the asparagus, bok choy, the radishes and the other ingredients, toss, cook for 12 minutes, divide between plates and serve.

Nutrition:

calories 140, fat 1, fiber 10, carbs 20, protein 8

Roasted Cauliflower and Broccoli

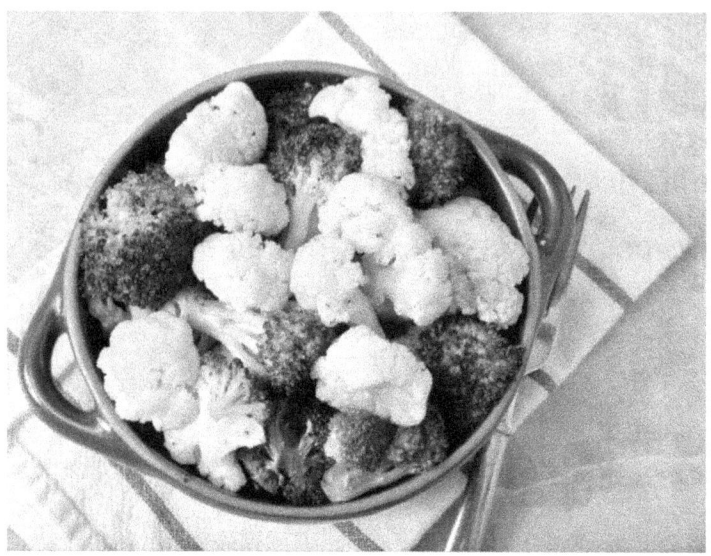

Preparation Time: 10 minutes

Cooking Time: 15 minutes

Servings: 12

Ingredients:

- 4 cups broccoli, florets
- 4 cups cauliflower, florets
- 6 cloves garlic, minced
- 1/3 cup extra-virgin olive oil
- 2/3 cup Parmesan cheese, grated, divided

- Pepper and salt to taste

Directions:

1. Preheat Your Oven To 450° Fahrenheit. Spray With Cooking Spray A Baking Dish, Then Set It Aside.
2. Add Broccoli, Cauliflower, Half Of The Cheese, Garlic, And Olive Oil Into A Mixing Bowl And Toss Well To Blend.
3. Season With Salt And Pepper. Arrange Cauliflower And Broccoli Mixture In Your Prepared Baking Dish.
4. Bake For 15 Minutes In Preheated Oven. Just Before Serving Add Remaining Cheese On Top.
5. Serve Hot And Enjoy!

Nutritional Values (Per Serving):

Calories: 81 Carbohydrates: 3.1 G Fat: 6.7 G Sugar: 1.1 G Cholesterol: 5 Mg Protein: 1.9 G

Mexican Vegan Mince

Preparation Time: 5 minutes

Cooking Time: 5 minutes

Serves: 4

Ingredients:

- 400 grams Seitan Mince
- 2 cloves Garlic, minced
- 2 pieces Green Chili, chopped
- 2 tbsp Nutritional Yeast
- 1 tbsp Garam Masala
- 1 tsp Cumin Powder
- 1 small Red Onion, diced
- 2 Roma Tomatoes, diced
- ½ tsp Salt
- Cilantro for garnish
- 2 tbsp Olive Oil

Directions:

1. Heat olive oil in a non-stick pan. Add onions, garlic, and green chili. Sautee until aromatic.

2. Add mince and stir-fry for 3-5 minutes.
3. Add nutritional yeast, garam masala, and cumin powder. Stir until well combined.
4. Season with salt to taste.
5. Garnish with fresh cilantro and serve.

Nutritional Values:

Kcal per serve: 232 Fat: 16 g. Protein: 17 g. Carbs: 9 g.

Chili-Garlic Edamame

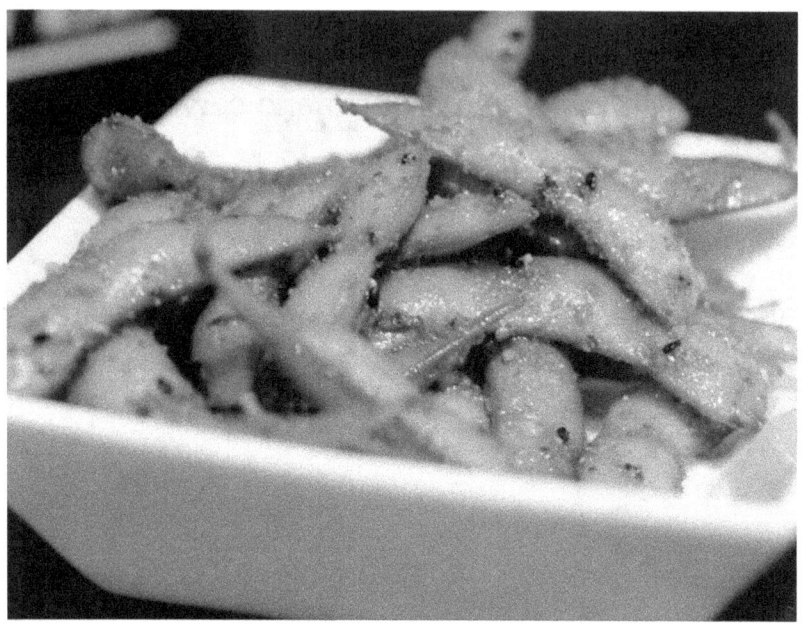

Preparation Time: 5 min

Cooking Time: 10 min

Serves: 4

Ingredients:

- 300 grams Edamame Pods
- 3 cloves Garlic, minced
- 1 tbsp Olive Oil

- ½ tsp Red Chili Flakes
- pinch of Salt

Directions:

1. Steam edamame for 5 minutes.
2. Heat olive oil in a pan.
3. Sautee garlic and chili until aromatic.
4. Add in steamed edamame and stir for a minute.
5. Season with salt.

Nutritional Values:

Kcal per serve: 126 Fat: 7 g. Protein: 8 g. Carbs: 8 g.

Arugugla Mushroom Salad

Preparation Time: 20 minutes

Servings: 4

Ingredients:

- 10 oz mushrooms, clean and cut the steam
- 4 cups arugula
- 2 tsp fresh rosemary, chopped
- 10 sun-dried tomatoes, chopped
- 2 garlic cloves, minced
- 1 tbsp vinegar
- 6 tbsp olive oil
- 1/2 tsp sea salt

Directions:

1. In a small bowl, combine together olive oil, vinegar, salt, rosemary, and garlic.
2. Add mushroom in a bowl, then pour olive oil mixture over mushrooms and set aside for 1 hour.

3. Preheat the oven to 480 °F.
4. Place mushrooms on rack and grill in preheated oven for 10 minutes.
5. Place arugula on the serving dish, then place grilled mushrooms and chopped tomatoes.
6. Serve and enjoy.

Nutritional Value (Amount per Serving):

Calories 261 Fat 22 g Carbohydrates 14 g Sugar 9 g Protein 5 g Cholesterol 0 mg

Spicy Cheese with Tofu Balls

Preparation Time: 20 minutes

Cooking Time: 20 minutes

Serving: 4

Ingredients:

For the spicy cheese:
- 1/3 cup vegan mayonnaise
- ¼ cup pickled jalapenos
- 1 tbsp mustard powder
- 1 tsp paprika powder
- 1 pinch cayenne pepper
- 4 oz grated tofu cheese

For the tofu balls:
- 1 tbsp flax seed powder + 3 tbsp water
- 2 ½ cup crumbled tofu
- 2 tbsp plant butter, for frying
- Salt and black pepper

Directions:

1. Make the spicy cheese. In a bowl, mix the mayonnaise, jalapenos, paprika, mustard powder, cayenne powder, and cheddar cheese. Set aside.
2. In another medium bowl, combine the flax seed powder with water and allow absorption for 5 minutes.
3. Add the flax egg to the cheese mixture, the crumbled tofu, salt, and black pepper, and combine well. Use your hands to form large meatballs out of the mix.
4. Then, melt the butter in a large skillet over medium heat and fry the tofu balls until cooked and browned on the outside.
5. Serve the tofu balls with roasted cauliflower mash and mayonnaise.

Nutrition:

Calories: 259, Total Fat: 55.9g, Saturated Fat:11.4 g, Total Carbs: 5 g, Dietary Fiber: 1g, Sugar: 1g, Protein: 16g, Sodium: 452mg

Cucumber and Cauliflower Mix

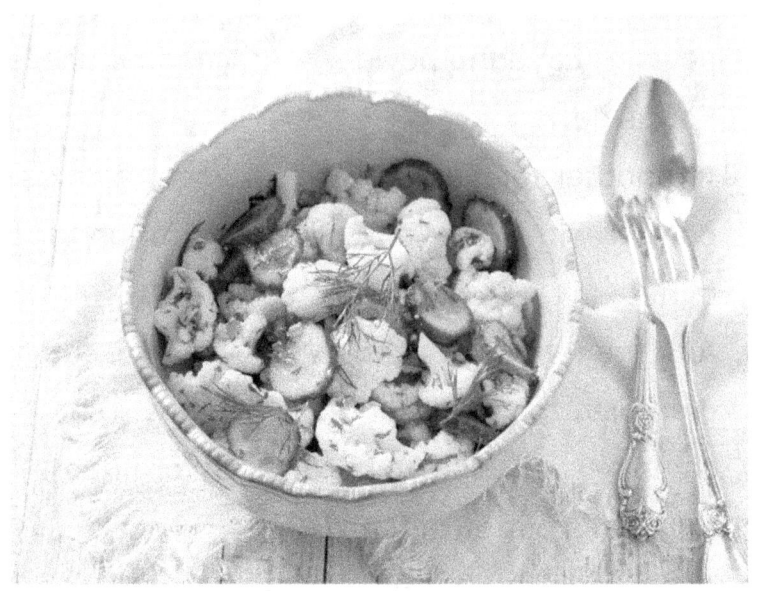

Preparation time: 10 minutes

Cooking time: 12 minutes

Servings: 4

Ingredients:

- 1 cucumber, cubed
- 1 spring onion, chopped
- 1 pound cauliflower florets
- 2 tablespoons avocado oil

- ¼ teaspoon red pepper flakes
- 1 tablespoon balsamic vinegar
- Salt and black pepper to the taste
- 1 tablespoon thyme, chopped

Directions:

1. Heat up a pan with the oil over medium heat, add the spring onions and the pepper flakes and sauté for 2 minutes.
2. Add the cucumber and the other ingredients, toss, cook over medium heat for 10 minutes more, divide between plates and serve.

Nutrition:

calories 53, fat 1.2, fiber 3.9, carbs 9.9, protein 3

Bell Pepper Sauté

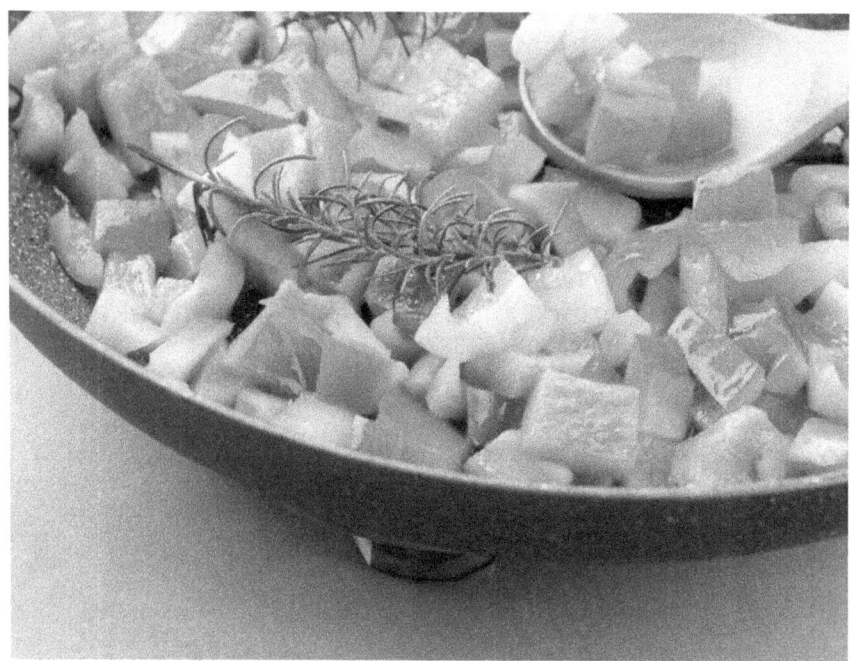

Preparation time: 5 minutes

Cooking time: 20 minutes

Servings: 4

Ingredients:

- 1 green bell pepper, cut into strips
- 1 red bell pepper, cut into strips
- 1 yellow bell pepper, cut into strips

- 1 orange bell pepper, cut into strips
- 3 scallions, chopped
- 1 tablespoon coconut aminos
- 1 tablespoon olive oil
- A pinch of salt and black pepper
- 1 tablespoon parsley, chopped
- 1 tablespoon rosemary, chopped

Directions:

1. Heat up a pan with the oil over medium-high heat, add the scallions and sauté for 5 minutes.
2. Add the bell peppers and the other ingredients, toss, cook over medium heat for 15 minutes more, divide between plates and serve.

Nutrition:

calories 120, fat 1, fiber 2, carbs 7, protein 6

Wild Rice Mix

Preparation time: 10 minutes

Cooking time: 6 hours

Servings: 12

Ingredients:

- 40 ounces veggie stock
- 2 and ½ cups wild rice
- 4 ounces mushrooms, sliced
- 1 cup carrot, shredded
- 2 tablespoons olive oil
- 2 teaspoons marjoram, dried and crushed
- 2/3 cup dried cherries
- ½ cup pecans, toasted and chopped
- 2/3 cup green onions, chopped
- Salt and black pepper to the taste

Directions:

1. In your slow cooker, mix stock with wild rice, carrot, mushrooms, oil, marjoram, salt, pepper, cherries, pecans and green onions, toss, cover and cook on Low for 6 hours.

2. Stir wild rice one more time, divide between plates and serve as a side dish.
3. Enjoy!

Nutrition:

calories 169, fat 5, fiber 3, carbs 28, protein 5

Squash And Spinach Mix

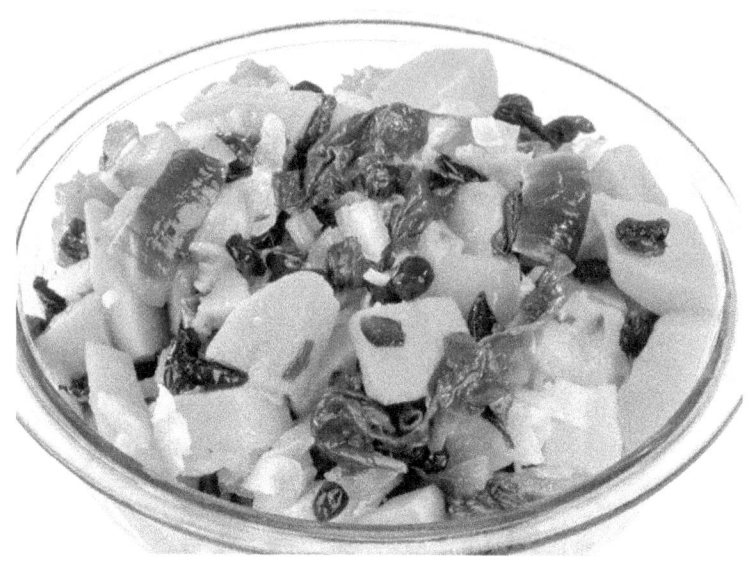

Preparation time: 10 minutes

Cooking time: 3 hours and 30 minutes

Servings: 12

Ingredients:

- 10 ounces spinach, torn
- 2 pounds butternut squash, peeled and cubed
- 1 yellow onion, chopped
- 1 cup barley

- 14 ounces veggie stock
- ½ cup water
- A pinch of salt and black pepper to the taste
- 3 garlic cloves, minced

Directions:

1. In your slow cooker, mix squash with spinach, barley, onion, stock, water, salt, pepper and garlic, toss, cover and cook on High for 3 hours and 30 minutes.
2. Divide squash mix on plates and serve as a side dish.
3. Enjoy!

Nutrition:

calories 196, fat 3, fiber 7, carbs 36, protein 7

Baked Artichokes and Green Beans

Preparation time: 10 minutes

Cooking time: 40 minutes

Servings: 4

Ingredients:

- 1 pound green beans, trimmed and halved
- 1 cup canned artichoke hearts, drained and quartered
- 3 scallions, chopped
- 2 tablespoons olive oil
- 2 garlic cloves, minced
- 1/3 cup tomato passata
- 2 teaspoons mustard powder
- 1 teaspoon cumin, ground
- A pinch of salt and black pepper
- 1 teaspoon coriander, ground

Directions:

1. Heat up a pan with the oil over medium heat, add the scallions and the garlic and sauté for 5 minutes.

2. Add the green beans and the other ingredients, toss, introduce in the oven and bake at 390 degrees F for 35 minutes.
3. Divide the mix between plates and serve as a side dish.

Nutrition:

calories 132, fat 7.8, fiber 6.9, carbs 14.8, protein 4.4

Herbed Risotto

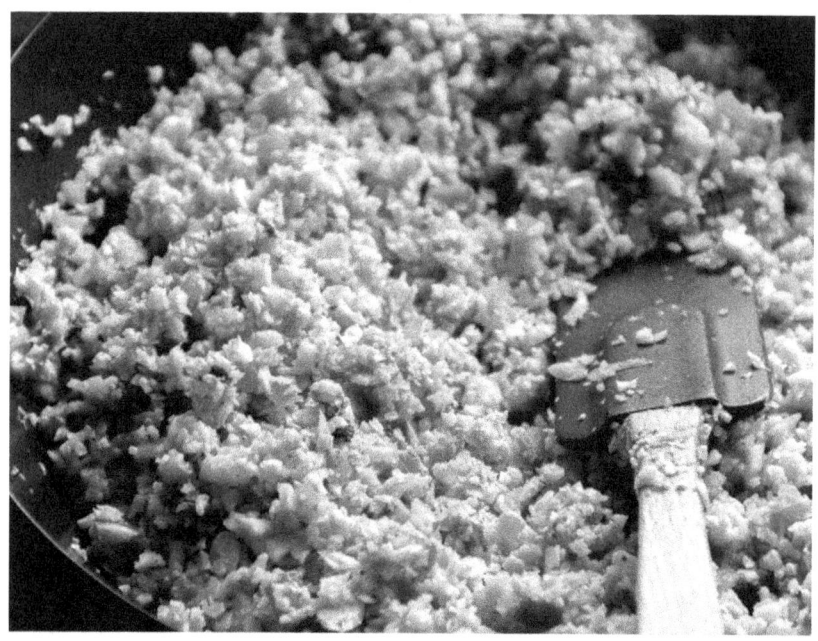

Preparation time: 10 minutes

Cooking time: 25 minutes

Servings: 4

Ingredients:

- 4 scallions, chopped
- 2 cups cauliflower rice
- 2 tablespoons avocado oil

- 2 cups veggie stock
- 1 tablespoon parsley, chopped
- 1 tablespoon cilantro, chopped
- 1 tablespoon basil, chopped
- Juice of 1 lime
- 1 tablespoon oregano, chopped
- 1 teaspoon sweet paprika
- A pinch of salt and black pepper

Directions:

1. Heat up a pan with the oil over medium heat, add the scallions and sauté for 5 minutes.
2. Add the cauliflower rice, the stock and the other ingredients, toss, cook over medium heat for 20 minutes, divide between plates and serve as a side dish.

Nutrition:

calories 182, fat 4, fiber 2, carbs 8, protein 10

Braised Cabbage And Apples

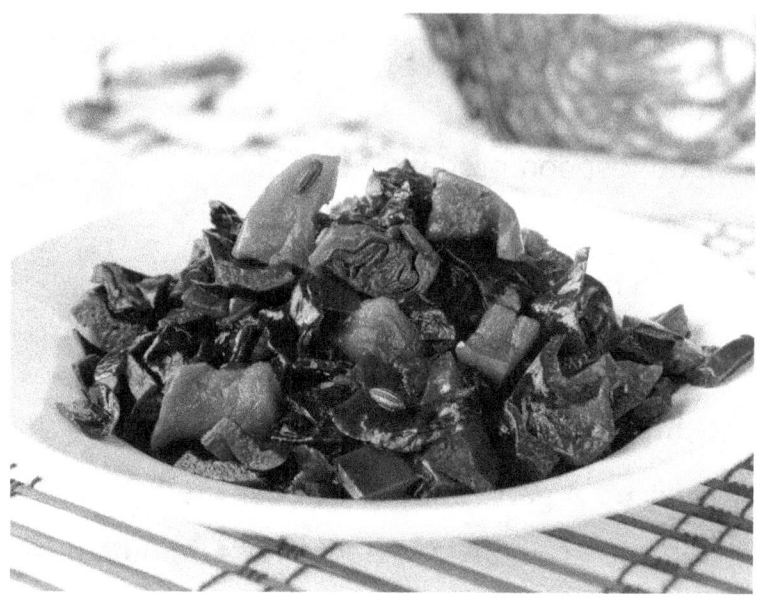

Preparation time: 5 minutes

cooking time: 25 minutes

servings: 6

Ingredients

- 2 tablespoons olive oil
- 1 Granny Smith apple
- 1 small head red cabbage, shredded
- 1 small head savoy cabbage, shredded

- 1 red cooking apple, such as Rome or Gala
- 2 tablespoons sugar
- 1/4 cup cider vinegar
- 1 cup water
- Salt and freshly ground black pepper

Directions

1. In a large saucepan, heat the oil over medium heat.
2. Add the shredded red and savoy cabbage, cover, and cook until slightly wilted, 5 minutes.
3. Core the apples and cut them into 1/4-inch dice.
4. Add the apples to the cabbage, along with the sugar, water, vinegar, and salt and pepper to taste.
5. Reduce heat to low, cover, and simmer until the cabbage and apples are tender, frequently stirring, about 20 minutes.
6. Serve immediately.

Eggplant and Garlic Sauce

Preparation time: 10 minutes

Cooking time: 10 minutes

Servings: 4

Ingredients:

- 3 eggplants, cut into halves and thinly sliced
- 2 tablespoons avocado oil
- 2 garlic cloves, minced
- 1 red chili pepper, chopped
- 1 green onion stalk, chopped
- 1 tablespoon ginger, grated
- 1 tablespoon coconut aminos
- 1 tablespoon balsamic vinegar

Directions:

1. Heat up a pan with half of the oil over medium-high heat, add eggplant slices, cook for 2 minutes, flip, cook for 3 minutes more and transfer to a plate.

2. Heat up the pan with the rest of the oil over medium heat, add chili pepper, garlic, green onions, ginger, stir, and cook for 1 minute.
3. Return eggplant slices to the pan, stir and cook for 1 minute.
4. Add coconut aminos and vinegar, stir, divide between plates and serve.
5. Enjoy!

Nutritional value/serving:

calories 123, fat 1,7, fiber 15,2, carbs 26,7, protein 4,4

Warm Watercress Mix

Preparation time: 10 minutes

Cooking time: 10 minutes

Servings: 4

Ingredients:

- 1 pound watercress, chopped
- 1 small shallot, peeled, cooked and chopped
- 1 garlic clove, cut in halves
- ¼ cup olive oil
- ¼ cup hazelnuts, chopped
- Black pepper to taste
- ¼ cup pine nuts

Directions:

1. Heat up a pan with the oil over medium heat, add garlic clove halves, cook for 2 minutes and discard.
2. Heat up the pan with the garlic oil again over medium heat, add hazelnuts and pine nuts, stir and cook for 6 minutes.

3. Add shallots, black pepper to taste and watercress, stir, cook for 2 minutes, divide between plates and serve right away.
4. Enjoy!

Nutritional value/serving:

calories 220, fat 21,8, fiber 2,1, carbs 2,9, protein 5,3

Purple Carrot Mix

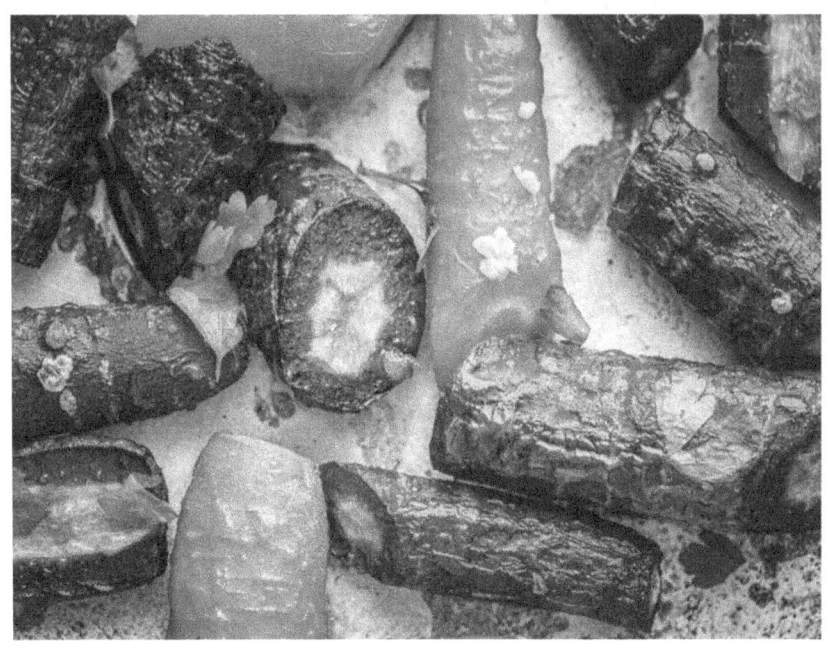

Preparation time: 10 minutes

Cooking time: 1 hour

Servings: 5

Ingredients:

- 6 purple carrots, peeled
- A drizzle of olive oil
- 2 tablespoons sesame seeds paste

- 6 tablespoons water
- 3 tablespoons lemon juice
- 1 garlic clove, minced
- Black pepper to taste
- A pinch of sea salt
- White sesame seeds for serving

Directions:

1. Arrange the purple carrots on a lined baking sheet, sprinkle a pinch of salt, black pepper and a drizzle of oil, place in the oven at 350 degrees F and bake for 1 hour.
2. Meanwhile, in a food processor, mix sesame seeds paste with water, lemon juice, garlic, a pinch of sea salt and black pepper and pulse well.
3. Spread over the carrots, toss gently, divide between plates and sprinkle sesame seeds on top.
4. Enjoy!

Nutritional value/serving:

calories 100, fat 4,7, fiber 0,9, carbs 13,6, protein 1,2

Broccoli, Garlic, and Rigatoni

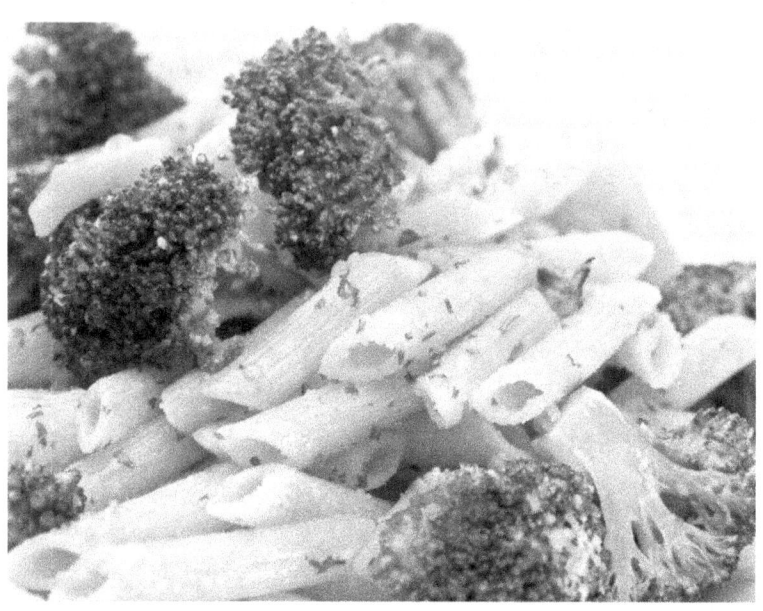

Preparation Time: 10 mins

Servings: 2

Ingredients:

- 2 tsps. Minced garlic
- 2 c. Broccoli florets
- 2 tbsps. Parmesan cheese
- Freshly ground black pepper
- 1/3 lb. Rigatoni noodles

- 2 tsps. Olive oil

Directions:

1. Fill a pot three-quarters of the way full with water and bring it to a boil. Add the rigatoni and cook until it is firm, around twelve minutes. Drain it thoroughly.
2. As the pasta cooks, bring an inch of water to a boil and put a steamer basket over the top.
3. Add the broccoli and steam for ten minutes.
4. In a bowl, mix together the pasta and broccoli. Toss with the cheese, oil, and garlic.
5. Season to taste and serve.

Nutrition:

Calories: 355, Fat:7 g, Carbs:63 g, Protein:14 g, Sugars:4 g, Sodium:600 mg

Broccoli Stew

Preparation time: 10 minutes

Cooking time: 40 minutes

Servings: 4

Ingredients:

- 1 broccoli head, separated into florets
- 2 teaspoons coriander seeds
- 1 onion, peeled and chopped
- A drizzle of olive oil
- Salt and ground black pepper, to taste
- A pinch of red pepper, crushed
- 1 small ginger piece, peeled, and chopped
- 1 garlic clove, peeled and minced
- 28 ounces canned pureed tomatoes

Directions:

1. Put water in a pot, add the salt, bring to a boil over medium-high heat, add the broccoli florets, steam them for 2 minutes, transfer them to a bowl filled with ice water, drain them, and leave aside.

2. Heat up a pan over medium-high heat, add the coriander seeds, toast them for 4 minutes, transfer to a grinder, ground them, and set aside as well.
3. Heat up a pot with the oil over medium heat, add the onions, salt, pepper, and red pepper, stir, and cook for 7 minutes.
4. Add the ginger, garlic, and coriander seeds, stir, and cook for 3 minutes.
5. Add the tomatoes, bring to a boil, and simmer for 10 minutes.
6. Add the broccoli, stir and cook the stew for 12 minutes.
7. Divide into bowls and serve.

Nutrition:

Calories - 150, Fat - 4, Fiber - 2, Carbs - 5, Protein - 12

Arugula Salad

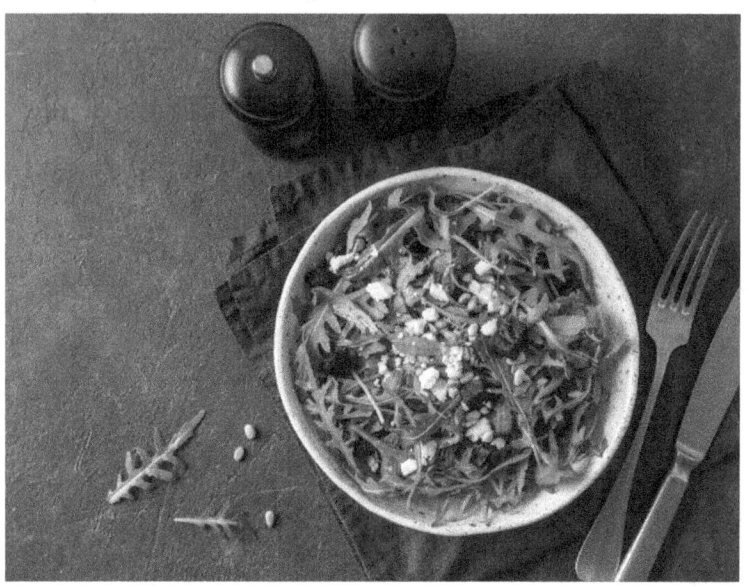

Preparation time: 10 minutes

Cooking time: 0 minutes

Servings: 4

Ingredients:

- 1 bunch baby arugula
- 1 white onion, peeled and chopped
- 1 tablespoon vinegar
- 1 cup hot water

- 2 tablespoons olive oil
- ¼ cup walnuts, chopped
- 2 tablespoons fresh cilantro, chopped
- 2 garlic cloves, peeled and minced
- Salt and ground black pepper, to taste
- 1 tablespoon lemon juice

Directions:

1. In a bowl, mix the water with vinegar, add the onion, set aside for 5 minutes, and drain well.
2. In a salad bowl, mix the arugula with the walnuts and onion, and stir.
3. Add the garlic, salt, pepper, lemon juice, cilantro, and oil, toss well, and serve.

Nutrition:

Calories - 200, Fat - 2, Fiber - 1, Carbs - 5, Protein - 7

Catalan-style Greens

Preparation time: 10 minutes

Cooking time: 15 minutes

Servings: 4

Ingredients:

- 1 apple, cored and chopped
- 1 onion, peeled and sliced
- 6 garlic cloves, peeled and chopped
- 3 tablespoons avocado oil
- ¼ cup raisins
- ¼ cup pine nuts, toasted
- ¼ cup balsamic vinegar
- 2½ cups Swiss chard
- 2½ cups spinach, and
- Salt and ground black pepper, to taste
- A pinch of nutmeg

Directions:

1. Heat up a pan with the oil over medium-high heat, add the onion, stir, and cook for 3 minutes.

2. Add the apple, stir, and cook for 4 minutes.
3. Add the garlic, stir, and cook for 1 minute.
4. Add the raisins, vinegar, spinach, and chard, stir, and cook for 5 minutes.
5. Add the nutmeg, salt, and pepper, stir, cook for a few seconds, divide on plates, and serve.

Nutrition:

Calories - 120, Fat - 1, Fiber - 2, Carbs - 3, Protein - 6

White And Wild Mushroom Barley Soup

Preparation time: 5 minutes

cooking time: 50 minutes

servings: 4 to 6

Ingredients

- 12 ounces white mushrooms, lightly rinsed, patted dry, and sliced
- 1 tablespoon olive oil
- 1 medium onion, chopped
- 1 medium carrot, chopped
- 2 celery ribs, chopped
- 8 ounces cremini, shiitake, or other wild mushrooms, lightly rinsed, patted dry, and cut into 1/4-inch slices
- 1 cup pearl barley
- 7 cups vegetable or mushroom broth, homemade (see Light Vegetable Broth or Mushroom Vegetable Broth or store-bought, or water
- 1 teaspoon dried dillweed
- Salt and freshly ground black pepper
- 2 tablespoons minced fresh parsley

Directions

1. In a large soup pot, heat the oil over medium heat. Add the onion, carrot, and celery.
2. Cover and cook until soft, about 10 minutes.
3. Uncover and stir in the mushrooms, barley, broth, dillweed, and salt and pepper to taste.
4. Bring to a boil, then reduce heat to low and simmer, uncovered, until the barley and vegetables are tender, about 40 minutes.
5. Add the parsley, taste, adjust seasonings if necessary, and serve.

Thai-Inspired Coconut Soup

Preparation time: 5 minutes

cooking time: 25 minutes

servings: 4

Ingredients

- 1 tablespoon canola or grapeseed oil
- 1 medium onion, chopped
- 2 tablespoons soy sauce
- 2 tablespoons minced fresh ginger
- 1 tablespoon light brown sugar (optional)
- 1 teaspoon Asian chili paste
- 21/2 cups light vegetable broth, homemade (see Light Vegetable Broth or store-bought, or water
- 8 ounces extra-firm tofu, drained and cut into 1/2-inch dice
- 2 (13.5-ouncecans unsweetened coconut milk
- 1 tablespoon fresh lime juice
- 3 tablespoons chopped fresh cilantro, for garnish

Directions

1. In a large soup pot, heat the oil over medium heat. Add the onion and ginger and cook until softened, about 5 minutes.
2. Stir in the soy sauce, sugar, and chile paste.
3. Add the broth and bring to a boil.
4. Reduce heat to medium and simmer for 15 minutes.
5. Strain the broth and discard solids.
6. Return the broth to the pot over medium heat.
7. Add the tofu and stir in the coconut milk and lime juice.
8. Simmer 5 minutes longer to allow flavors to blend.
9. Ladle into bowls, sprinkle with cilantro, and serve.

Tofu Avocado Keto Noodles

Preparation Time: 15 minutes

Serving: 4

Ingredients:

- 2 tbsp butter
- 1 lb tofu
- 8 large red and yellow bell peppers, Blade A, noodles trimmed
- 1 tsp garlic powder
- Salt and black pepper to taste
- 2 medium avocados, pitted, peeled and mashed
- 2 tbsp chopped pecans for topping

Directions:

1. Melt the butter in a large skillet and cook the tofu until brown, 5 minutes. Season with salt and black pepper.
2. Stir in the bell peppers, garlic powder and cook until the peppers are slightly tender, 2 minutes.

3. Mix in the mashed avocados, adjust the taste with salt and black pepper and cook for 1 minute.
4. Dish the food onto serving plates, garnish with the pecans and serve warm.

Nutrition:

Calories:209, Total Fat:15.2g, Saturated Fat:7.3g, Total Carbs:8g, Dietary Fiber:1g, Sugar:2g, Protein:13g, Sodium:468mg

Crunchy Cauliflower Bites

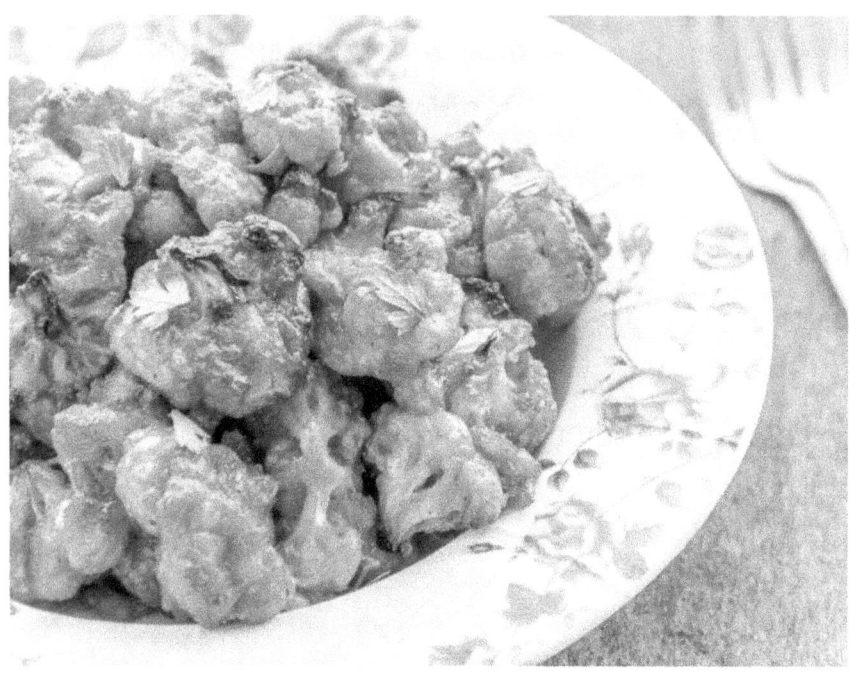

Preparation Time: 10 minutes

Cooking Time: 20 minutes

Servings: 8

Ingredients:

- 2 eggs, organic, beaten
- ½ head cauliflower, cut into florets
- 1 tablespoon Parmesan cheese, grated

- 1 cup breadcrumbs
- Pepper and salt to taste

Directions:

1. Preheat your oven to 395°Fahrenheit. Spray baking dish with cooking spray and set aside.
2. In a shallow dish combine the cheese, breadcrumbs, pepper, and salt.
3. Dip the cauliflower florets in beaten egg then roll in breadcrumb mixture.
4. Place coated cauliflower florets onto the prepared baking dish.
5. Bake in preheated oven for 20 minutes.
6. Serve hot and enjoy!

Nutrition:

Calories: 81 Sugar: 1.3 g Fat: 2.4 g Carbohydrates: 10.7 g Cholesterol: 42 mg Protein: 4.3 g

Broccoli and Almonds

Preparation Time: 5 minutes

Cooking Time: 12 minutes

Servings: 4

Ingredients:

- 1 lb. broccoli florets
- ½ cup almonds; chopped
- 1 tbsp. chives; chopped
- 3 garlic cloves; minced
- 2 tbsp. red vinegar
- 3 tbsp. coconut oil; melted
- A pinch of salt and black pepper

Directions:

1. Take a bowl and mix the broccoli with the garlic, salt, pepper, vinegar and the oil and toss.
2. Put the broccoli in your air fryer's basket and cook at 380 °F for 12 minutes
3. Divide between plates and serve with almonds and chives sprinkled on top.

Nutrition:

Calories: 180 Fat: 4g Fiber: 2g Carbs: 4g Protein: 6g

Twice Baked Spaghetti Squash

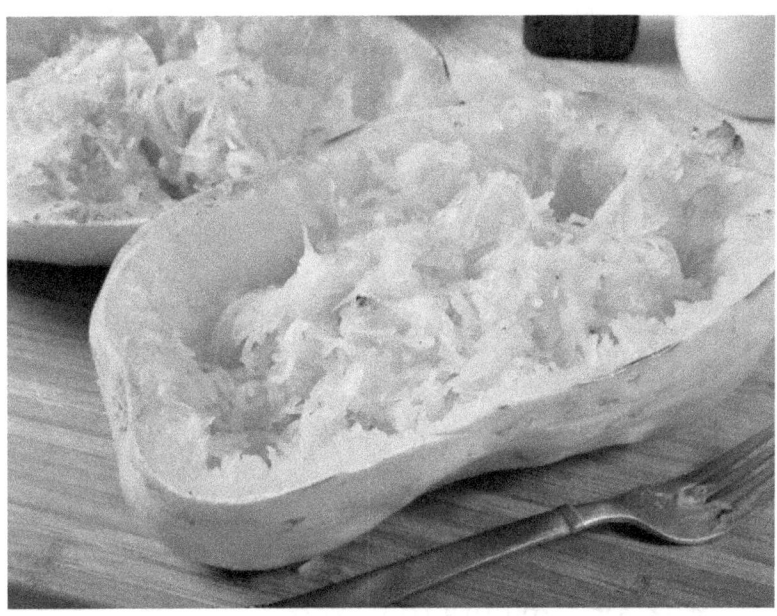

Preparation Time: 15 minutes

Cooking Time: 55 minutes

Servings: 6

Ingredients:

- 2pounds spaghetti squash
- ¾ cup pecorino romano cheese, shredded (or parmesan)
- 1 tablespoon olive oil

- 1 cup mozzarella cheese, shredded
- 1 tablespoon butter
- 1 teaspoon onion powder
- 2 tablespoons fresh thyme leaves
- 3 cloves garlic, minced
- ½ teaspoon salt
- ¼ teaspoon pepper

Directions:

1. Preheat oven to 400 °F.
2. Use a fork to poke a few holes around the spaghetti squash. Put in the microwave and cook for a minute to soften a bit.
3. On a cutting board, cut off the end of squash, then cut in half lengthwise. Use a spoon to scrape the pulp and seeds. Rub inside surface with olive oil.
4. Place each piece of squash, cut side down, onto the baking sheet.
5. Bake 40-50 minutes or until it has become fork tender.
6. Let cool for a bit and then use a fork to remove all the strands of spaghetti squash into a mixing bowl.

7. Put pecorino romano cheese and mozzarella cheese into small dish then add HALF the cheese mixture to the bowl with squash.
8. Add butter, minced garlic, onion powder, fresh thyme, salt and pepper.
9. Using a fork, mash and mix thoroughly to combine everything with the squash flesh.
10. Spoon this squash mixture back into the skins on a baking sheet pan.
11. Sprinkle tops with the rest of the cheese mixture and return to oven.
12. Broil 5-6 minutes or until the cheese is melted and starting to brown.
13. Serve hot.

Nutrition:

Calories: 173, Total Fats: 12g, Carbohydrates: 10g, Fiber: 2g

Spicy Jalapeno Brussels sprouts

Preparation Time: 5 minutes

Cooking Time: 10 minutes

Servings: 4

Ingredients:

- 1 lb Brussels sprouts
- 1 jalapeno pepper, seeded and chopped
- 1 medium onion, chopped
- 1 tbsp olive oil
- Pepper
- Salt

Directions:

1. Heat olive oil in a pan over medium heat.
2. Add onion and jalapeno in the pan and sauté until softened.
3. Add Brussels sprouts and stir until golden brown, about 10 minutes.
4. Season with pepper and salt.
5. Serve and enjoy.

Nutrition:

Calories 91, Fat 3.9g, Carbohydrates 13.1g, Sugar 3.7g, Protein 4.2g, Cholesterol 0mg

Risotto Bites

Preparation time: 15 minutes

cooking time: 20 minutes

servings: 12 bites

Ingredients

- ½ cup panko bread crumbs
- 1 teaspoon paprika
- 1½ cups cold Green Pea Risotto
- 1 teaspoon chipotle powder or ground cayenne pepper
- Non-stick cooking spray

Directions

1. Preheat the oven to 425 ºF.
2. Line a baking sheet with parchment paper.
3. On a large plate, combine the panko, paprika, and chipotle powder. Set aside.
4. Roll 2 tablespoons of the risotto into a ball.
5. Gently roll in the bread crumbs and place on the prepared baking sheet. Repeat to make a total of 12 balls.

6. Spritz the tops of the risotto bites with nonstick cooking spray and bake for 15 to 20 minutes, until they begin to brown.
7. Cool completely before storing in a large airtight container in a single layer (add a piece of parchment paper for a second layer or in a plastic freezer bag).

Nutrition (6 bites):

Calories: 100; Fat: 2g; Protein: 6g; Carbohydrates: 17g; Fiber: 5g; Sugar: 2g; Sodium: 165mg

Jicama and Guacamole

Preparation time: 15 minutes

cooking time: 0 minutes

servings: 4

Ingredients

- 2 hass avocados, peeled, pits removed, and cut into cubes
- juice of 1 lime, or 1 tablespoon prepared lime juice
- ½ teaspoon sea salt
- ½ red onion, minced
- 1 garlic clove, minced
- ¼ cup chopped cilantro (optional
- 1 jicama bulb, peeled and cut into matchsticks

Directions

1. In a medium bowl, squeeze the lime juice over the top of the avocado and sprinkle with salt.
2. Lightly mash the avocado with a fork.

3. Stir in the onion, garlic, and cilantro, if using.
4. Serve with slices of jicama to dip in guacamole.
5. To store, place plastic wrap over the bowl of guacamole and refrigerate.
6. The guacamole will keep for about 2 days.

Black Sesame Wonton Chips

Preparation time: 5 minutes

cooking time: 5 minutes

servings: 24 chips

Ingredients

- 12 Vegan Wonton Wrappers
- Toasted sesame oil
- 1/3 cup black sesame seeds
- Salt

Directions

1. Preheat the oven to 450 °F. Lightly oil a baking sheet and set aside. Cut the wonton wrappers in half crosswise, brush them with sesame oil, and arrange them in a single layer on the prepared baking sheet.
2. Sprinkle wonton wrappers with the sesame seeds and salt to taste, and bake until crisp and golden brown, 5 to 7 minutes. Cool completely before serving. These are best eaten on the day they are made but, once cooled, they can be covered and stored at room temperature for 1 to 2 days.

Peppers and Hummus

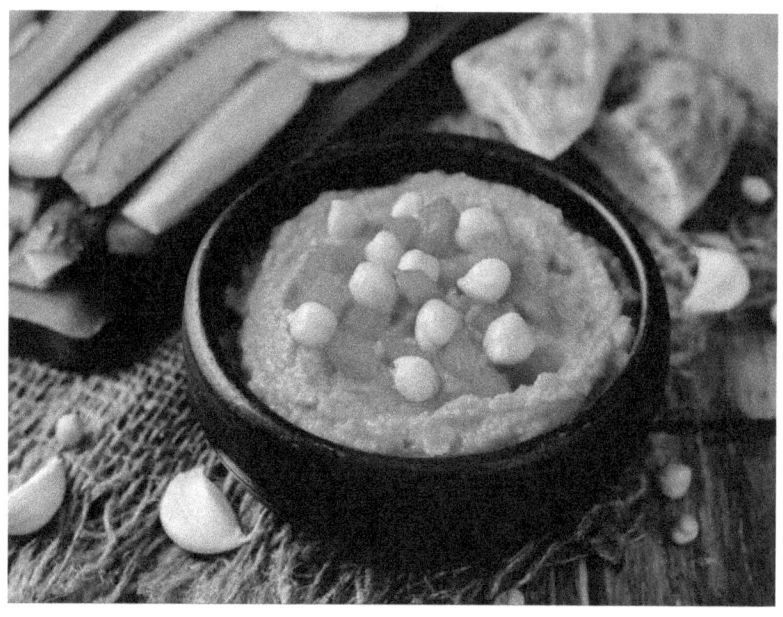

Preparation time: 15 minutes

cooking time: 0 minutes

servings: 4

Ingredients

- one 15-ounce can chickpeas, drained and rinsed
- juice of 1 lemon, or 1 tablespoon prepared lemon juice
- ¼ cup tahini

- 3 tablespoons olive oil
- ½ teaspoon ground cumin
- 1 tablespoon water
- ¼ teaspoon paprika
- 1 red bell pepper, sliced
- 1 green bell pepper, sliced
- 1 orange bell pepper, sliced

Directions

1. In a food processor, combine chickpeas, lemon juice, tahini, 2 tablespoons of the olive oil, the cumin, and water.
2. Process on high speed until blended, about 30 seconds.
3. Scoop the hummus into a bowl and drizzle with the remaining tablespoon of olive oil.
4. Sprinkle with paprika and serve with sliced bell peppers.

Crispy Brussels Sprouts

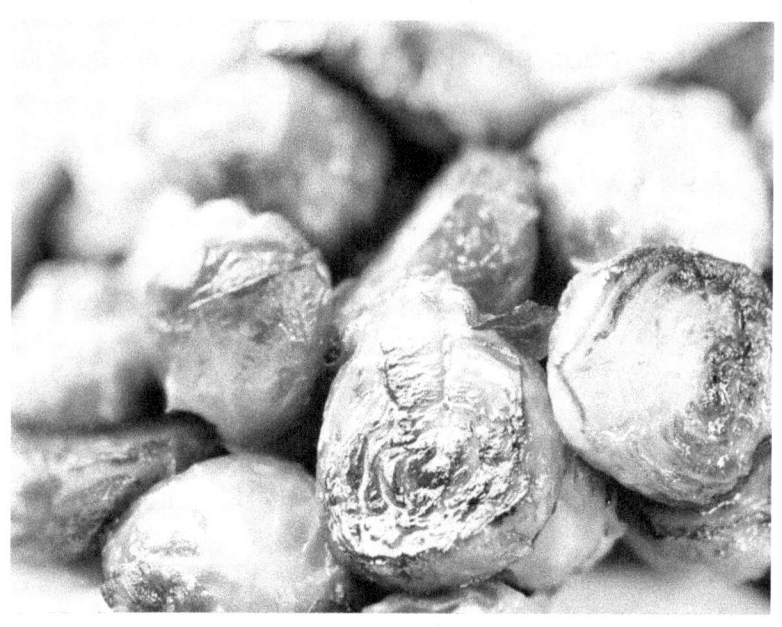

Preparation time: 10 minutes

Cooking time: 30 minutes

Servings: 4

Ingredients:

- 2 pounds Brussels sprouts, trimmed and halved
- 2 tablespoons avocado oil
- 1 teaspoon red pepper flakes
- 1 tablespoon smoked paprika

- 1 tablespoon balsamic vinegar
- A pinch of salt and black pepper

Directions:

1. In a roasting pan, combine the sprouts with the pepper flakes, paprika and the other ingredients, toss and cook at 400 degrees F for 30 minutes.
2. Divide the Brussels sprouts into bowls and serve as a snack.

Nutrition:

calories 162, fat 4, fiber 3, carbs 7, protein 8

Coconut Bites

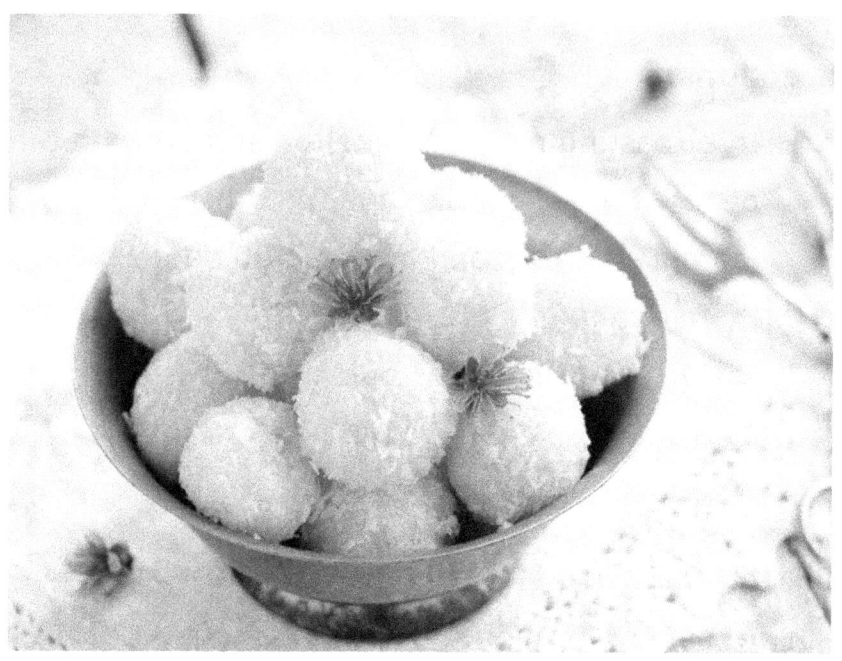

Preparation time: 10 minutes

Cooking time: 25 minutes

Servings: 6

Ingredients:

- 1 and ½ cup coconut flesh, unsweetened and shredded
- 1 cup coconut milk

- A pinch of salt
- ¼ cup chives, chopped
- 2 teaspoons rosemary, dried
- Cooking spray

Directions:

1. In a pan, combine the coconut with the coconut milk and the other ingredients except the cooking sp ray, whisk and cook over medium heat for 10 minutes.
2. Take spoonfuls of this mix, shape medium balls, arrange them all on a baking sheet lined with parchment paper, grease them with the cooking spray, and cook at 450 degrees F for 15 minutes.
3. Serve the coconut bites cold.

Nutrition:

calories 112, fat 3, fiber 3, carbs 3, protein 8

Spiced Okra Bites

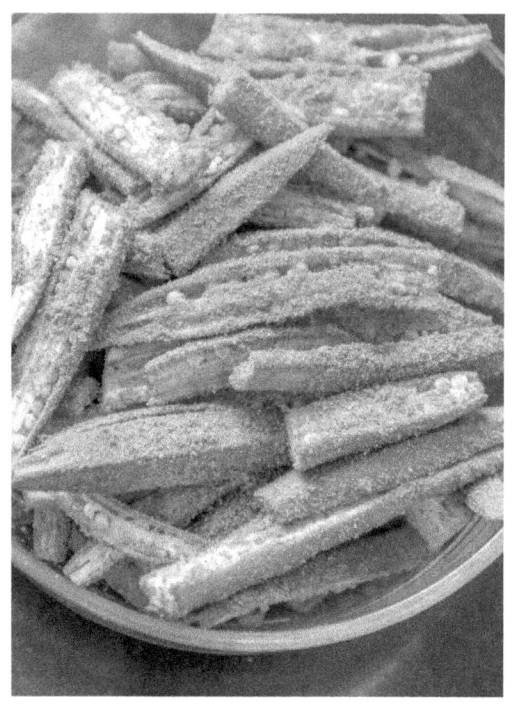

Preparation time: 10 minutes

Cooking time: 15 minutes

Servings: 4

Ingredients:

- 2 cups okra, sliced
- 2 tablespoons avocado oil

- ¼ teaspoon mustard powder
- ¼ teaspoon chili powder
- ¼ teaspoon garlic powder
- ¼ teaspoon onion powder
- A pinch of salt and black pepper

Directions:

1. Spread the okra on a baking sheet lined with parchment paper, add the oil and the other ingredients, toss and roast at 400 degrees F for 15 minutes.
2. Divide the okra into bowls and serve as a snack.

Nutrition:

calories 200, fat 2, fiber 2, carbs 6, protein 7

Chaffle Cannoli

Preparation Time: 15 minutes

Cooking Time: 28 minutes

Servings: 4

Ingredients:

For the chaffles:

- 1 large egg
- 1 egg yolk
- 1 tbso swerve confectioner's
- 3 tbsp butter, melted
- 1 cup finely grated Parmesan cheese
- 2 tbsp finely grated mozzarella cheese

For the cannoli filling:

- ½ cup ricotta cheese
- 2 tbsp swerve confectioner's sugar
- 1 tsp vanilla extract
- 2 tbsp unsweetened chocolate chips for garnishing

Directions:

1. Preheat the cast iron pan.
2. Meanwhile, in a medium bowl, mix all the ingredients for the chaffles.
3. Open the iron, pour in a quarter of the mixture, cover, and cook until crispy, 7 minutes.
4. Remove the chaffle onto a plate and make 3 more with the remaining batter.
5. Meanwhile, for the cannoli filling:
6. Beat the ricotta cheese and swerve confectioner's sugar until smooth. Mix in the vanilla.
7. On each chaffle, spread some of the filling and wrap over.
8. Garnish the creamy ends with some chocolate chips.
9. Serve immediately.

Nutrition:

Calories 308, Fats 25.05g, Carbs 5.17g, Net Carbs 5.17g, Protein 15.18g

Mango Coconut Cream Pie

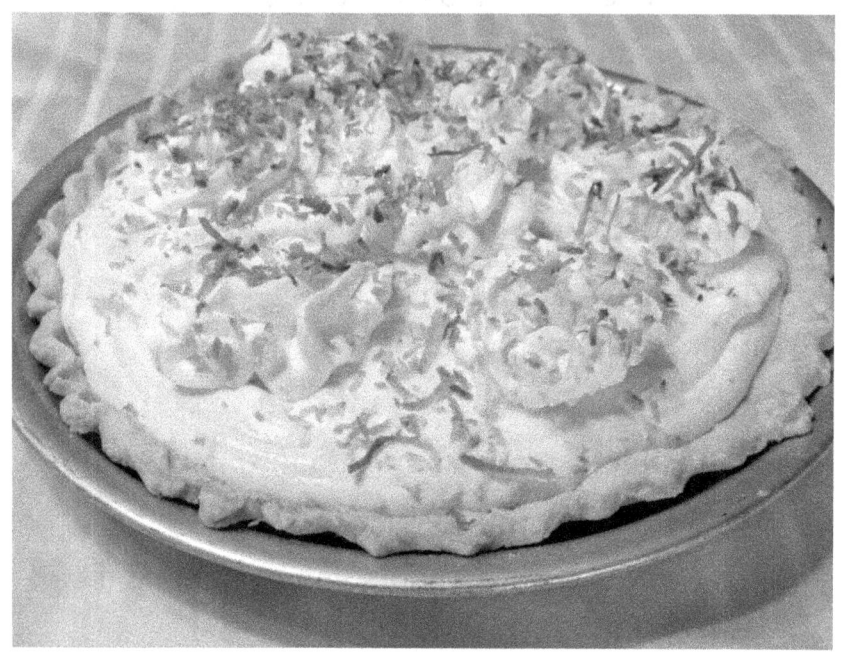

Preparation time: 20 minutes • chill time: 30 minutes servings: 8

Ingredients

For the crust

- ½ cup rolled oats
- 1 cup soft pitted dates
- 1 cup cashews

For the filling

- 1 cup canned coconut milk
- ½ cup water
- 2 large mangos, peeled and chopped, or about 2 cups frozen chunks
- ½ cup unsweetened shredded coconut

Directions

1. Put all the crust ingredients in a food processor and pulse until it holds together. If you don't have a food processor, chop everything as finely as possible and use ½ cup cashew or almond butter in place of half the cashews.
2. Press the mixture down firmly into an 8-inch pie or springform pan.
3. Put the all filling ingredients in a blender and purée until smooth (about 1 minute). It should be very thick, so you may have to stop and stir until it's smooth.
4. Pour the filling into the crust, use a rubber spatula to smooth the top, and put the pie in the freezer until set, about 30 minutes.
5. Once frozen, it should be set out for about 15 minutes to soften before serving.

6. Top with a batch of Coconut Whipped Cream scooped on top of the pie once it's set.
7. Finish it off with a sprinkling of toasted shredded coconut.

Nutrition (1 slice)

Calories: 427; Total fat: 28g; Carbs: 45g; Fiber: 6g; Protein: 8g

Lime in the Coconut Chia Pudding

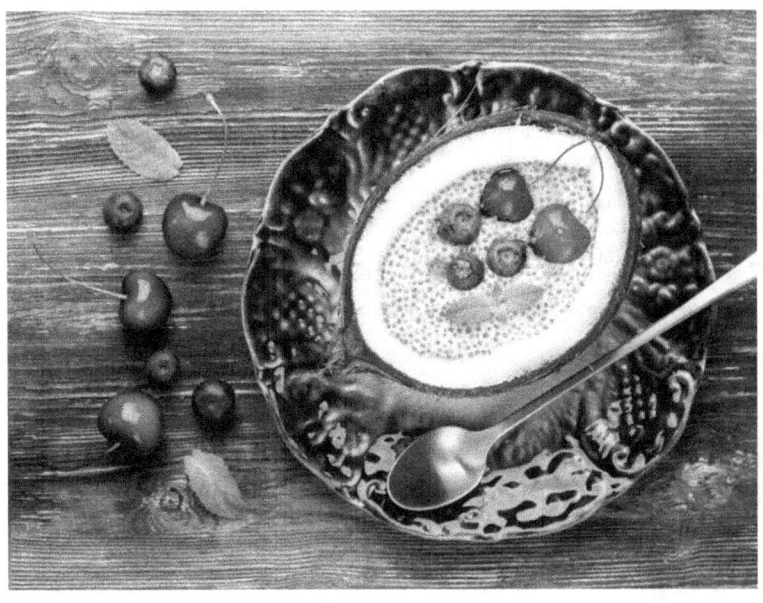

Preparation time: 10 minutes • chill time: 20 minutes

servings: 4

Ingredients

- Zest and juice of 1 lime
- 1 (14-ouncecan coconut milk
- 1 to 2 dates, or 1 tablespoon coconut or other unrefined sugar, or 1 tablespoon maple syrup, or 10 to 15 drops pure liquid stevia

- 2 tablespoons chia seeds, whole or ground
- 2 teaspoons matcha green tea powder (optional)

Directions

1. Blend all the ingredients in a blender until smooth.
2. Chill in the fridge for about 20 minutes, then serve topped with one or more of the topping ideas.
3. Try blueberries, blackberries, sliced strawberries, Coconut Whipped Cream, or toasted unsweetened coconut.

Nutrition

Calories: 226; Total fat: 20g; Carbs: 13g; Fiber: 5g; Protein: 3g

Grapefruit Cream

Preparation time: 10 minutes

Cooking time: 0 minutes

Servings: 4

Ingredients:

- 2 cups coconut cream
- 2 tablespoons stevia
- 1 cup grapefruit, peeled, and chopped
- 1 teaspoon vanilla extract

Directions:

1. In a blender, combine the coconut cream with the grapefruit and the other ingredients, pulse well, divide into bowls and serve cold.

Nutrition:

calories 346, fat 35.5, fiber 0, carbs 3.4, protein 4.6

Chia Bars

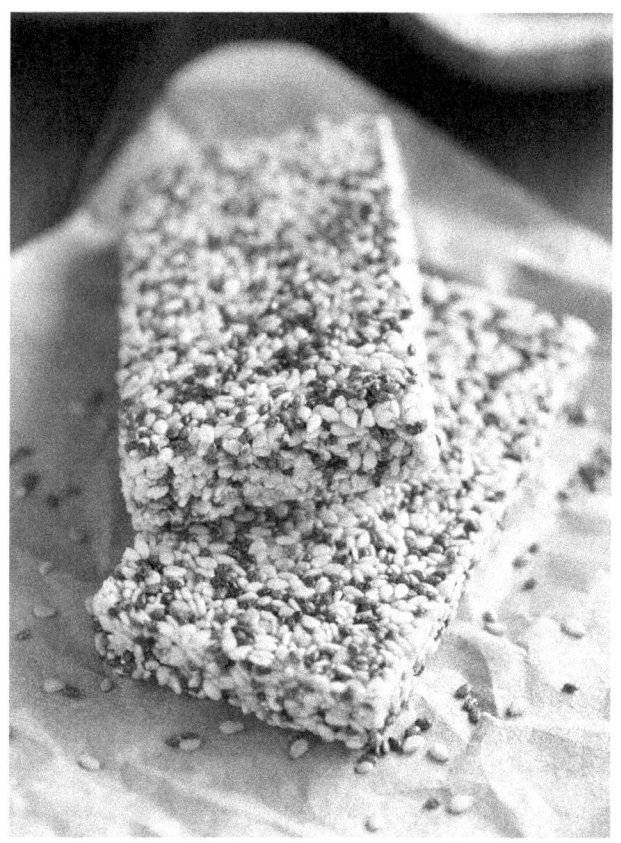

Preparation time: 10 minutes

Cooking time: 20 minutes

Servings: 6

Ingredients:

- 3 tablespoons chia seeds
- 1 cup coconut oil, melted
- ½ teaspoon baking soda
- 2 tablespoons stevia
- 1 cup coconut cream
- 3 tablespoons flaxseed mixed with 4 tablespoons water

Directions:

1. In a bowl, combine the coconut oil with the cream, the chia seeds and the other ingredients, whisk well, pour everything into a square baking dish, introduce in the oven at 370 degrees F and bake for 20 minutes.
2. Cool down, slice into squares and serve.

Nutrition:

calories 220, fat 2, fiber 0.5, carbs 2, protein 4

Fudgy Chocolate Cake

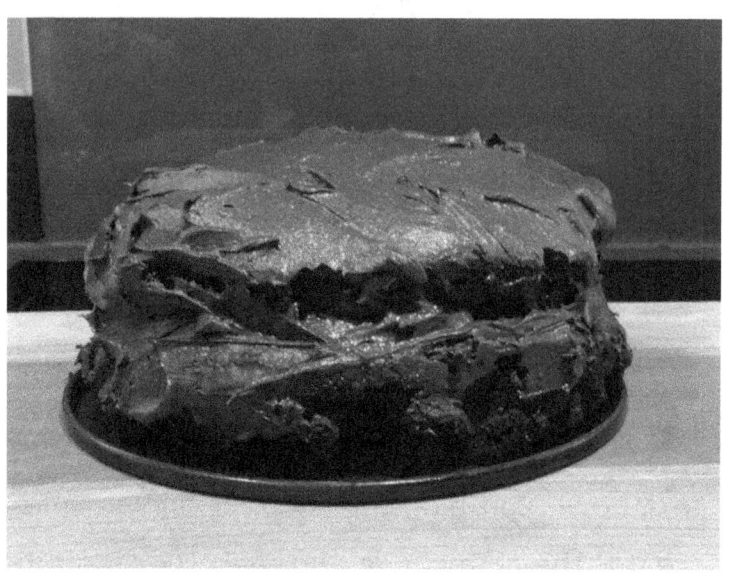

Preparation Time: 20 Minutes

Servings: 8

Ingredients:

Cake:

- 1½ cups unbleached all-purpose flour
- 2/3 cup granulated natural sugar
- 1 cup non-dairy milk
- ¼ cup unsweetened cocoa powder

- 3 tablespoons vegan butter, softened
- 1½ teaspoons baking powder
- 1 teaspoon pure vanilla extract
- ½ teaspoon cider vinegar
- ¼ teaspoon salt
- ¼ teaspoon baking soda

Frosting:

- 1½ cups confectioners' sugar, plus more if needed
- 2 tablespoons vegan butter, melted
- ¼ cup unsweetened cocoa powder
- 3 tablespoons non-dairy milk, plus more if needed
- 1 teaspoon pure vanilla extract

Directions:

1. Lightly oil a baking tray that will fit in the steamer basket of your Cooker.
2. In a bowl combine the flour, cocoa powder, baking soda, baking powder, and salt.
3. Whisk the vegan butter and granulated sugar until they form a creamy blend.
4. Add the milk, vinegar, and vanilla.

5. Add the flour mixture and stir until evenly mixed.
6. Pour the batter into your baking tray and put the tray in your steamer basket.
7. Pour the minimum amount of water into the base of your Cooker and lower the steamer basket.
8. Seal and cook on Steam for 12 minutes.
9. Release the pressure quickly and set to one side to cool a little.
10. For the frosting, stir the cocoa into the melted butter until smoothly blended.
11. Add the milk and vanilla and mix well again.
12. Stir in the sugar until you have an almost pourable frosting.
13. Refrigerate until it's time to frost your cake.

Baked Apples.

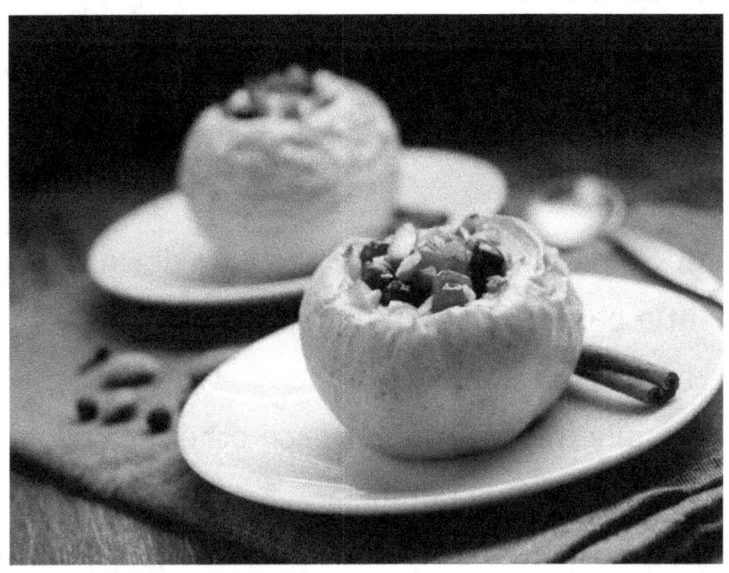

Preparation Time: 35 Minutes

Servings: 6

Ingredients:

- 6 large firm Granny Smith apples, washed
- ⅓ cup sweetened dried cranberries
- ½ cup naturally sweetened cranberry juice
- ⅓ cup packed light brown sugar or granulated natural sugar

- ¼ cup crushed, chopped, or coarsely ground almonds, walnuts, or pecans
- Juice of 1 lemon
- ½ teaspoon ground cinnamon

Directions:

1. Core the apples most of the way down, leaving a little base so the stuffing stays put.
2. Stand your apples upright in your Cooker. Do not pile them on top of each other! You may need to do two batches.
3. In a bowl combine the sugar, nuts, cranberries, and cinnamon.
4. Stuff each apple with the mix.
5. Pour the cranberry juice around the apples.
6. Seal and cook on Stew for 20 minutes.
7. Depressurize naturally.

Cream Cheese Cookies

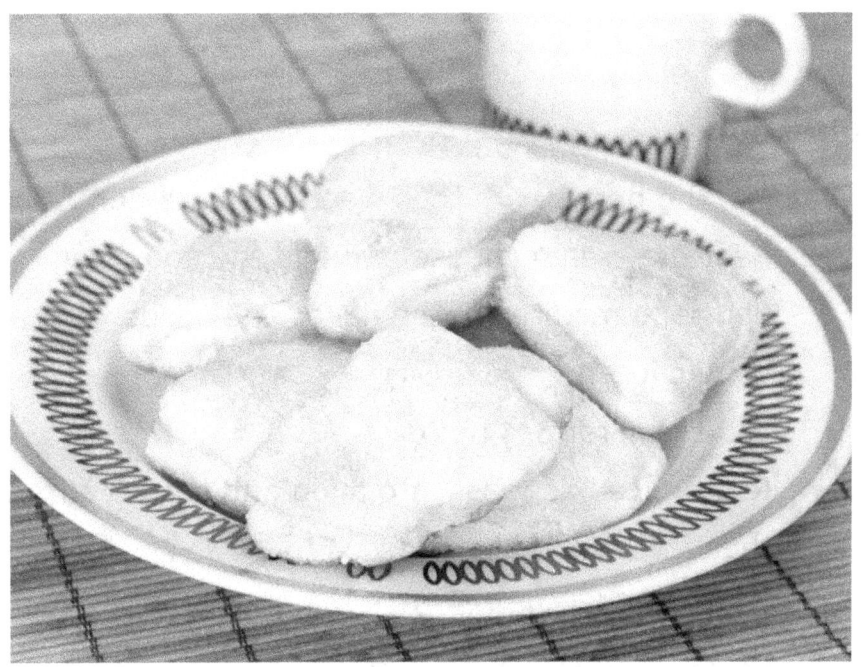

Preparation time: 40 minutes

Ingredients:

- 1 egg
- 1 cup butter
- ¾ cup stevia or any sugar substitute
- 4 Oz. cream cheese, softened
- 2 cups almond flour

- 1 cup coconut flour
- Sesame seeds
- Vanilla or any flavored extract to taste

Directions:

1. Mix the butter with the sweetener until fluffy.
2. Beat the cream cheese and add the egg, then flour and mix it with the flavor and seeds you have chosen.
3. Let it chill for 3-4 hours.
4. Roll the cookie mass into a log and have it sliced thus forming your cookies.
5. Bake until brown up to 15 minutes or more to make them crispy.

Yogurt Smoothie with Cinnamon and Mango

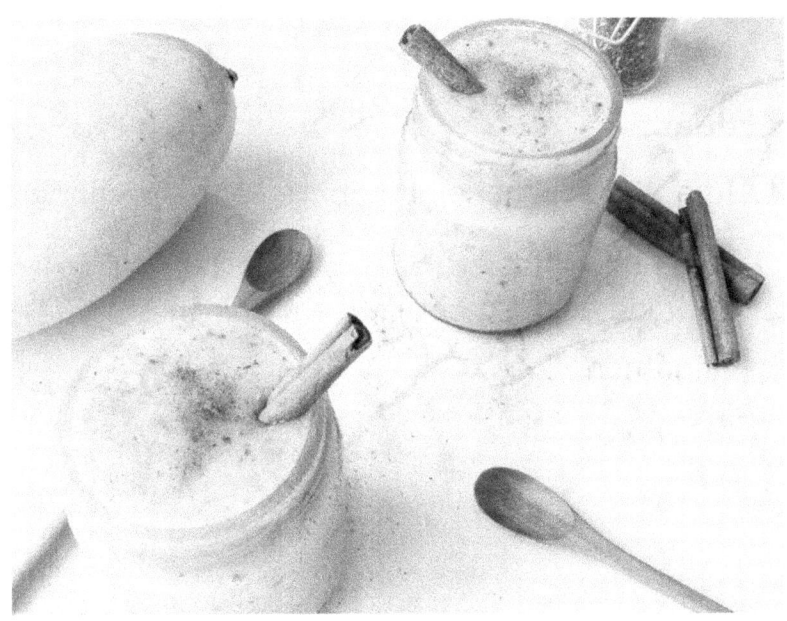

Preparation time: 15 minutes

Ingredients:

- 4 Oz. frozen mango chunks, mango pulp or fresh mango
- 1 cup Greek yogurt
- 1 cup coconut milk, full fat

- 3-4 cups milk
- 3 tbsp. flax seed meal
- 1 tbsp. honey
- 1 tsp. cinnamon

Directions:

1. In a blender mix all the ingredients, except cinnamon until smooth.
2. Sprinkle each smoothie with a pinch of cinnamon.

Cocoa Peach Cream

Preparation time: 10 minutes

Cooking time: 0 minutes

Servings: 4

Ingredients:

- 2 cups coconut cream
- 1/3 cup stevia
- ¾ cup cocoa powder
- Zest of 1 lime, grated
- 1 tablespoons lime juice
- 2 peaches, pitted and chopped

Directions:

1. In a blender, combine the cream with the stevia, the cocoa and the other ingredients, pulse well, divide into cups and serve cold.

Nutrition:

calories 172, fat 5.6, fiber 3.5, carbs 7.6, protein 4

Minty Almond Cups

Preparation time: 10 minutes

Cooking time: 10 minutes

Servings: 4

Ingredients:

- 1 cup almonds, roughly chopped
- 1 tablespoon mint, chopped
- ½ cup coconut cream
- 2 tablespoons stevia
- 1 teaspoon vanilla extract

Directions:

1. In a pan, combine the almonds with the mint, the cream and the other ingredients, whisk, simmer over medium heat for 10 minutes, divide into cups and serve cold.

Nutrition:

calories 135, fat 4.1, fiber 3.8, carbs 4.1, protein 2.3

Lime Cake

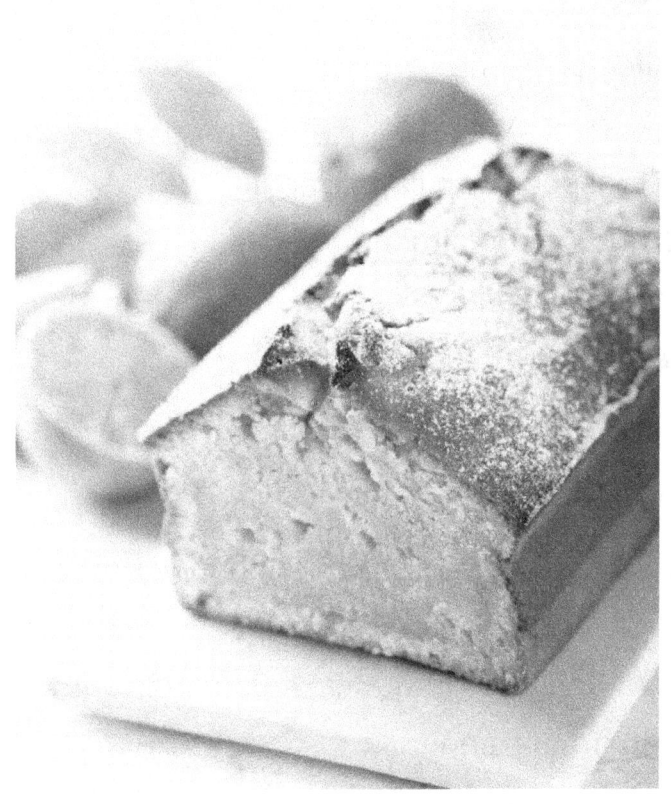

Preparation time: 10 minutes

Cooking time: 40 minutes

Servings: 4

Ingredients:

- ½ cup almonds, chopped
- Zest of 1 lime grated
- 2 tablespoons flaxseed mixed with 3 tablespoons water
- Juice of 1 lime
- 1 cups stevia
- 1 teaspoon vanilla extract
- 1 and ½ cup almond flour
- ½ cup coconut cream
- 1 teaspoon baking soda

Directions:

1. In a bowl, combine the almond with the lime zest, lime juice and the other ingredients, whisk well and pour into a cake pan lined with parchment paper.
2. Introduce in the oven at 360 degrees F, bake for 40 minutes, cool down, slice and serve.

Nutrition:

calories 186, fat 16.4, fiber 3, carbs 6.8, protein 4.7

Berry Cream

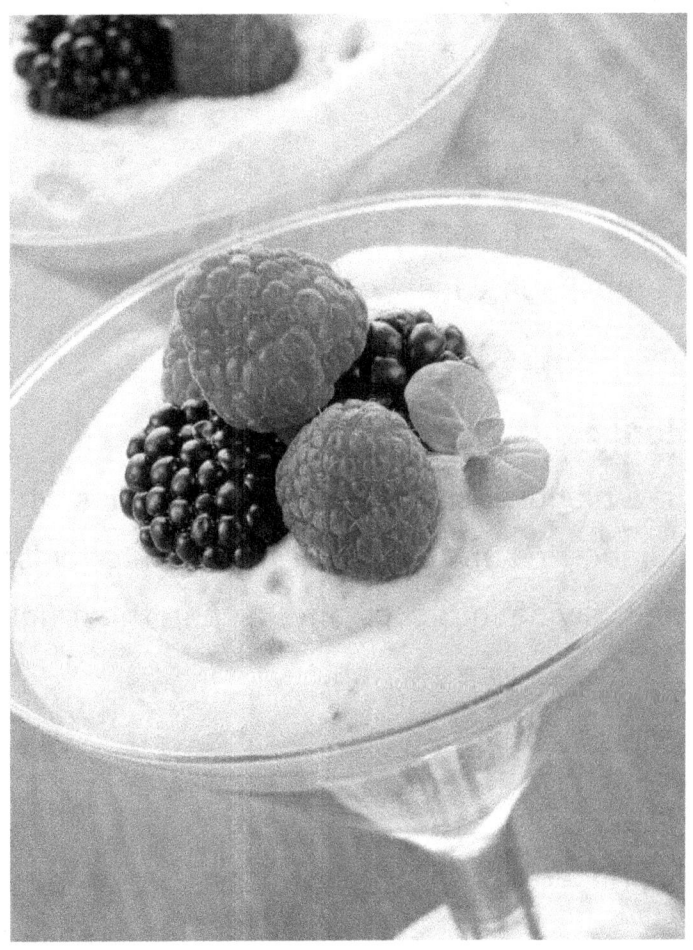

Preparation time: 2 hours

Cooking time: 0 minutes

Servings: 4

Ingredients:

- 1 cup strawberries, chopped
- 1 cup blueberries
- 1 cup coconut cream
- 1/3 cup stevia
- 1 teaspoon lime juice
- ¼ teaspoon nutmeg, ground
- ½ teaspoon vanilla extract

Directions:

1. In a blender, combine the strawberries with the blueberries and the other ingredients, pulse well, divide into cups and keep in the fridge for 2 hours before serving.

Nutrition:

calories 200, fat 4.5, fiber 3.3, carbs 5.6, protein 3.4

NOTE

www.ingramcontent.com/pod-product-compliance
Lightning Source LLC
Chambersburg PA
CBHW070102120526
44589CB00033B/1510